Imn Boosters:

How to Naturally Boost Your Immune System and Stay Healthy All Year Long

A Month-by-Month Guide Featuring Immunity Strengthening Herbs, Natural Antibiotics, Essential Oils, Gut Healthy Nutrition and Holistic Living Strategies

By Mary Thibodeau

Copyright © 2015, by Mary Thibodeau. All rights reserved. No part of this publication may be reproduced, distributed, or transmitted in any form or by any means, including photocopying, recording, or other electronic or mechanical methods, without the prior written permission of the publisher, except in the case of brief quotations embodied in critical reviews and certain other noncommercial uses permitted by copyright law.

Disclaimer: This book is not intended as a substitute for the medical advice of your health care practitioner. The reader should regularly consult a physician in matters relating to his/her health and diet, and particularly with respect to any symptoms that may require diagnosis or medical attention.

Table of Contents

Introduction

January - Get The Ball Rolling - 5 Immunity Hacks

February's Favorite - Vitamin C

March - Food To Fuel Your Immune System

April - Effective Natural Cleansing

May - Enhancing Brain Function For Immunity

June - Personal Empowerment & Immunity

July - Deep Internal Healing With Calendula

August - Using Essential Oils For Optimal Immunity

September - Fermented Foods For Immunity

October - Winter Preparation Month #1

November - Winter Preparation Month #2

December - 6 Delicious Immunity Recipes

Bonus Recipe - One Last Immunity Booster

Conclusion

References

Introduction

I am not a doctor. I did not spend years learning about immunity in a higher educational setting and I don't try to pretend that I did. What I have come to know about our immune system through daily living is that the things I do can directly affect how I feel and how often I get sick.

We as humans are surrounded by and often immersed in potentially harmful microorganisms. Potentially is the key word. If our immune system is functioning properly it provides our body with its own effective defense mechanism.

Our immune system responds the same way to whatever threat it faces: first it identifies foreign substances, then it isolates them and prevents them from spreading. When it's working the way nature intended, the job gets done and we stay healthy.

So what happens when for some reason the immunity system is compromised? I don't mean when we're faced with a virus or bacterial infection. Our immune system has specific needs in order to function as intended. Let's take a look at a few of the most important requirements:

1. Just like every other system in our body, the immune system needs the right FUEL for all its working parts. When we eat a meal that we know is truly awful and devoid of nutritional value, we are not just creating a problem for our digestive system to handle. We are depriving our whole body of the fuel it needs to thrive, including our immunity system.

2. Not getting enough SLEEP does not just make us tired, it robs our bodies of time to heal and regenerate, across all bodily systems.

3. STRESS does not just affect our nervous system; it affects all systems, including our immunity. People who have undergone extreme stress can attest to the direct correlation between stressful situations and health. Plentiful medical studies back it up.

Many of us, by minimizing or ignoring these basic physiological needs for adequate fuel, rest and reduced stress, will end up enduring a lot more sickness. We have compromised our immunity so we're not only sicker more often, *but we've made it harder to get better*.

There are many ways we can boost our immunity system, give it more of what it needs and enhance its ability to work for our health. In the following chapters you'll find a thorough rundown of dozens of holistic ways to help your immune system really work for you.

If you google 'immunity', the first website that comes up is the U.S. government's website, www.vaccine.gov. But when I think of natural immunity I just do not think of vaccines. To me that is *un*natural immunity. And I know I'm putting myself out there to take a lot of flack for that statement, but over the years of self study and practicing natural health methods, I have come to discover that you can naturally make yourself healthier.

You have the ability to improve your chances against disease in ways that are holistic, side effect free, and that actually benefit you in a multitude of ways.

In the U.S. today this is widely understood yet grossly ignored. Why? Mainly because of habit. We have grown used to taking a pill to make a symptom go away. It's easy and fast and if there are problems, well, there are more pills and procedures to back you up.

I wrote this book because we cannot live an energetic and dynamic lifestyle if we depend only on vaccines and other pharmaceuticals for health because they simply cannot bring it on their own. So, what does bring it?

Paying special attention to our immunity system in relation to all other body systems and naturally supporting our bodies with:

~Immunity Strengthening Herbs
~Natural Antibiotics
~Gut Healthy Nutrition
~Holistic Living Strategies

In this book I'm going to show you how to take your immunity into your own hands with all natural strategies, including techniques I have spent over a decade studying, observing and implementing on my family and myself. I want each person that reads this to know that they can make a huge difference in their own health by building up their immunity naturally. I want people to know that our immunity system is amazingly adept at fighting disease - all we need to do is provide it with the right tools.

January - Get The Ball Rolling

I'm starting my immunity book with the month of January because I feel this is the crucial month for natural health. After the holidays and the rush and the gorging, we are left with a long winter ahead. Especially in the colder regions, what you do in this long, dark and cold month will either carry you through the rest of the winter, or drag you down into sickness and fatigue.

I believe firmly that if you can TAKE January, just kill January with extra natural health practices, you are going to thrive, and when spring comes you will be better than ever. That is the goal of caring for your immunity system in January.

Here are my top 5 January Immunity Hacks:

January Immunity Hack# 1 - Schizandra (Schisandra chinensis)
This is the perfect herb to talk about when discussing Holistic Health. What do I mean by Holistic? Well in this book I am focusing on natural immunity. But we cannot increase our immunity as a separate entity, apart from, say our cardiovascular or nervous systems. Your body's self defense mechanism is dependent on the health of all your body parts and they in

turn cannot function optimally without a healthy immune system.

That's why I always prefer the holistic route as opposed to our modern day "allopathic" medical model. Allopathic medicine treats a symptom and works to eliminate that symptom. Holistic medicine looks at the body as a whole and recognizes symptoms as signals of distress; messages for us to sit up and take notice. Suppressing a symptom without getting to root of the distress is a temporary measure.

When we value holistic medicine, we're able to take a close look at our overall health and optimize everything. I hope this makes sense to those of you who are new to holistic medicine.

So, back to Schizandra; I placed this herb in the #1 spot in the first chapter of this book for a reason:

This lovely berry, eaten raw, dried and used in teas, capsules or as a tincture, provides the following benefits to a human body:

-Regulates and normalizes blood sugar
-Acts a an anti-inflammatory
-Is a mind tonic; aids in memory, concentration and intellectual activity
-Is an adaptogenic, meaning it can bring your body from an extreme state (such as in depression, or sickness) to a balanced state.

-Promotes healthy cellular function with strong antioxidant properties
-Balances central nervous system, easing anxiety
-Purifies the blood with its liver cleansing capacities and acts as a powerful detoxifier
-Repairs liver tissues and protects against fatty liver degeneration
-Nourishes and tones the respiratory system
-Its natural astringents are known for rejuvenating skin, thus being associated with preserving a youthful glow
-Relieves coughs and congestion
-Tones urinary tract system
-Brings reproductive system into balance and increases libido
-Combats stress with its calming effects while also producing mental clarity (with no jitters)
-Increases stamina and endurance
-Aids with insomnia
-Nourishes the heart and cardiovascular system

Basically, outside of reattaching a severed limb or performing brain surgery, Schizandra pretty much does it all. And the all is what you want - support your immunity by bringing your body back into balance in the first place.

Schizandra has been used and considered THE premium herb for health for THOUSANDS of years. While our current medical system is dominated by symptom suppressing and problem causing pharmaceuticals, this ancient knowledge is readily available to us now. Read below for five simple ways to include this powerhouse herb in your daily life:

Five Easy Ways To Take Schizandra:

1-Eat the berries. You will hear this time and time again from me when reading my books. If you want the power of the herb, if it can be eaten fresh, do it. If you can go outside and forage for these berries and have them fresh to eat, in my opinion there is no better way. (This is not the case with all herbs, though, many are better dried or otherwise prepared when used for medicine, and others may even be toxic if eaten. But in the case of Schizandra berries, they are both a healthy food and medicine.)

2-Take the tincture. This is the 2nd best option because tinctures are usually made with the fresh herb and are preserved, almost indefinitely - usually in alcohol because this extracts more medicine than glycerin or apple cider vinegar. It's also easy to just take 10 drops per day under the tongue. If you don't like the taste of the alcohol, you can also put the drops into your morning tea, or any hot beverage for that matter, and the alcohol will either be diluted or burn off so the taste of it is limited. However, you do have a higher absorption rate when the medicine is taken under the tongue, as opposed to being drunk and digested.

3-In a tea. You can dry your own berries or buy them from a natural food store or online source and make a nice cup of tea with 1-2 teaspoons of the dried berries and steeping for 15-20 minutes.

4-Take capsules. Usually taking 2 capsules per day, each with about 1 gram of the dried herb, is suggested. My concern here is that sometimes there are preservatives in with the herb; other times the herb may have been sprayed at some point with pesticides, especially if not organic. The fresher the better, so finding a local source or a reputed organic source will help you get the best quality Schizandra Berries available.

5-In a fruit smoothie. You can grind up the dried berries first in a coffee grinder, or if you have a powerful smoothie blender, that should do the trick. This makes a great way to soup up your breakfast. If you have fresh berries, these can be used as well.

January Immunity Hack #2 - Hydrate
We all know that humans can go several weeks without food, but we will not survive many days without water. If you're wondering what water has to do with immunity, here are five reasons our bodies need proper hydration to stay healthy:

1-Having enough water ensures that our blood is oxygenated.

2-Water is necessary in digesting and eliminating food.
3-Proper hydration means toxins are readily flushed out.
4-More water will help you sleep better since it's required to produce melatonin.
5-Adequate water means our mouth and eyes are moist, which they need to be in order to do their jobs: repelling germs, dirt, dust, etc.

Drinking water to improve immunity may sound overly simple to you, but I literally could write an entire book about the benefits of hydration. Adequate water for our bodily systems is vital in January because:

-The Heat. If you live in a non tropical place, you are going to have the heat on. And heat dries. I watch the heat dry my wet laundry quicker than the hot sun. I see my indoor plants' need for water drastically increase as soon as it's cold enough to turn on the heat.

-The Lacks. Most of us are lacking in January; we've seen a reduction in fresh air, sunshine, exercise and the availability of fresh foods.

Getting your 8 cups a day will ensure that your immune system is functioning optimally because:

a. Drinking copious amounts of water increases blood oxygenation, enhancing the workings of all bodily systems; and assists the kidneys in removing waste from your body

b. It keeps your digestion moving along properly so that needed nutrients can get where they need to go - to all the cells in your body.

c. January can be a depressing month and I can tell you without a doubt in my mind that having enough water heightens your mood. Your whole body will feel good and your energy reserves will be spent less on trying to function, and more on repair and reinvigoration.

d. The more water you drink, the better your ability to produce lymph, the transporter of white blood cells and nutrients to all your bodily tissues.

So how do you get enough water? Here's 5 tips:

1-Drink two cups first thing upon waking

2-Make your breakfast a huge fruit smoothie

3-Eat only fruit for breakfast (or any other meal) - citrus fruits and melons are full of water and vitamin C = win/win. Try 8 tangerines, or a 6 banana smoothie with blueberries.

4-Make a pot of ginger tea in the morning and drink it all day long

5-Steam Inhalations or lots of baths and showers. You can boil water, pour into a large bowl adding a few drops of pure Eucalyptus Essential Oil (another herbal antibiotic) and wrap yourself in the steam with a towel for 15 minutes. This provides extra moisture to your mouth, nose and eyes which are the essential germ catchers, and especially needed during the cold and flu season. Extras baths and showers can garner you the same results.

January Immunity Hack #3 - Eat Turnips
You heard me right, turnips!! Did you know that this lowly root vegetable is a powerful and nutrient-packed immunity buster? How is this possible? It is possible because turnips are full of the things your immune system needs for functioning.

For one, Vitamin B6 - Scientists have studied the effects of B6 deficiency (which is common in the western world) and concluded that not getting enough B6 can result in:

-Decreased immune response
-Impaired ability to produce antibodies
-A negative change in tumor growth

Two cups of steamed, mashed turnip provide about 25% of your daily requirement of B6.

(Nuts and seeds are also excellent sources as well as bananas and avocados).

That same serving of turnips will also garner you over 70% of your daily Vitamin C and a wide range of other vitamins and minerals including Vitamin K (an antioxidant), Vitamin A (helps cell growth and immunity), and potassium and magnesium, just to name a few.

If you are able to get the turnip _greens_ tossed into the mix, you are now talking even more fiber as well these nutrients:

471% Vitamin A
53% Vitamin C
42% Folate
588% Vitamin K
40% Copper
27% Manganese
etc. etc. the list goes on!!

I love it when I can spread the word about healthy food. Food that not only fills up your belly and tastes good, but food that gives you the most bang for your buck, economically as well as nutritionally. Including turnips as a staple in your winter diet can boost your overall health and immunity.

To help you ease into your new turnip habit, here are 3 creative and easy ways to prepare these humble root veggies:

Baked Root Medley
Ingredients:
- 1 large turnip, peeled and cubed
- 2 small boiling potatoes, halved
- 1 large sweet potato, peeled and cubed
- 2 large parsnips, peeled and cubed
- 2 large carrots, peeled and cubed
- 3 tablespoons olive oil
- 3 tablespoons sweet red chili sauce
- 1 large onion, chopped
- 1 1/2 teaspoons garlic powder
- 1 teaspoon ground black pepper
- 1 teaspoon cayenne
- Preheat oven to 375 degrees F (190 degrees C).

Directions:
- Toss potatoes, turnip, sweet potato, parsnips, onion and carrots with olive oil and chili sauce in a large bowl until coated. Season with garlic powder, cayenne, and pepper. Toss again until evenly coated, then spread vegetables into a 9x13 inch roasting pan.
- Roast vegetables in preheated oven for 20 minutes, then stir, return to oven, and continue cooking until the vegetables are tender, about 20 minutes more.

Sauteed Turnips With Turnip Greens
Peel 2-3 turnips, and slice thinly. Cook with 2 garlic cloves sliced in 2 tablespoons of olive oil

in a large skillet until tender. Add the turnip greens and cook until just wilted. Season with salt and pepper and a squeeze of lemon juice.

Spicy Mashed Turnips
Peel and slice 2 large turnips and steam until fork tender (may take 20-30 minutes depending on the thickness of the slices). Mash and add 1 teaspoon each of thyme and parsley (either dried or fresh), 1 teaspoon minced garlic, ¼ cup of rice or almond milk, a dash of ginger and salt and pepper to taste.

January Immunity Hack #4 - Vitamin D
If you haven't started supplementing with Vitamin D yet, now is the time. By January, our built up reserves of this immunity supporting vitamin are seriously depleted.

We've had the fact that Vitamin D is essential for bones driven into our brains for years, but its importance to our immunity system is now gaining attention as studies have repeatedly revealed that Vitamin D deficiency increases your susceptibility to infection.

In fact, Vitamin D deficiency is prevalent in autoimmune diseases such as Rheumatoid Arthritis, Graves Disease, Lupus and Ulcerative Colitis. Having a sufficient amount of D influences our adaptive and innate immune responses, meaning our immunity cells respond directly to Vitamin D, helping our system produce antibacterial, infection-fighting peptides.

How do you know if you are Vitamin D deficient? If you answer yes to any of the questions below, it's more likely than not that you are Vitamin D deficient:

-Is your skin dark?
-Are you depressed?
-Are you over 50 years old?
-Do weigh more than 30 pounds over your ideal weight?
-Are you experiencing fatigue with achiness?
-Do you live in a northern latitude, or above the 37th parallel? To get an idea, Richmond, Virginia and San Francisco are both just above this invisible line.
-Do you fracture easy or have weak muscles?

Now you know I am always recommending food choices for nutritional balance, and indeed, Vitamin D can be found in many foods, like eggs, salmon, liver and mushrooms. That doesn't leave a whole lot of choices if you're a vegan like me! And mushrooms, while certainly they can be nutritious and delicious - well, let's just say you'd have to eat 20 servings in one day to get 100IU of Vitamin D! Adding them to your diet can give you a little extra Vitamin D, as well as many other vitamins and minerals, but it's not a realistic strategy for D supplementation.

Vitamin D can also be found in fortified cereals and milk. But this type of vitamin D is harder for our body to synthesize so taking a vitamin supplement is generally preferred.

So with food sources not a workable option, supplementation of some kind is necessary, if you are unable to get the right amount of sunshine all year long. The recommended daily amount (though this can vary, ask your healthcare practitioner) is 600IU of Vitamin D3 or even more, since no adverse effects have been noted in patients taking up to 10,000IU per day. Basically, if you are deficient, you can take more.

If you want to find out exactly how deficient you are, you can get a blood test through your doctor. But if you live above that 37th parallel, I would go ahead and assume you need more D and start supplementing right away.

January Immunity Hack # 5 - Heat Up Your Metabolism

It's easy to sit around snuggled with a book and a blanket during this frosty month. But the more you do that, the colder cold you will feel in general. I'm not saying to stop reading and snuggling! But by incorporating this one tip into your winter routine, you can stay warmer all day from the inside out and even sleep better. What's the answer?

Exercise in the morning.

I'm not talking about waking up and immediately start running. Your body needs a little time adjusting to your waking state (and I have tips about maximizing that in an upcoming chapter!) But I have spent 47 winters in Maine and without a doubt, the very best winter days are those that include morning exercise.

I remember one winter when I was living near an abandoned railroad track. Each morning before going to work, I would go cross country skiing for 30 minutes on the trail the old tracks provided for me. Not only was that invigorating and enjoyable, but it kept me warm at my sedentary office job throughout the day. Stimulating your metabolism in this way gets it going - gets it off to a great start and keeps you warmer for longer. I have also found that exercising early increases my chances of getting in <u>more</u> fitness activities throughout the day because I feel more energy overall.

It doesn't have to be cross country skiing. This morning I was lacking in time and just did 50 jumping jacks. Believe it or not, that will be help keep me feeling warmer during my day and also helps me stay motivated to exercise more. This has a huge influence on your immunity. Here's why:

-In a study with cancer patients, those taking a 12-week exercise class were shown to exhibit enhanced T-cell production. Another study revealed that women who exercised the most, had the least risk of breast cancer.

-Exercise triggers Increased circulation and heart efficiency, so your body can do a better job of carrying blood, nutrients, hormones and waste products.

-Your respiratory system will have enhanced capabilities when it comes to oxygenating your blood and all your cells.

-The efficiency of your body's bacteria-fighting cells is increased, so they work faster.

I hope you enjoyed January's immunity hacks and have made it through that long dark month. Next up, in February, we'll talk about one of our immune system's most necessary nutrients.

February's Favorite: Vitamin C

Even if you were only able to incorporate one of January's immunity hacks, you should be in a better position to handle the deep winter month of February. At this point, we've been dealing with winter for a few months and have hopefully acclimated to the colder weather a bit. But many people during this time start to really see their health break down. So much time spent inside with drying heat and the lack of sun can wear a body down. It's time to look at really giving our immune system a well-needed boost.

So this month we will focus on Vitamin C, what it does, how much you need, and how to get it.

What it does:
Vitamin C's main functions are to assist in the repair and regeneration of bodily tissues, aid in the absorption of iron, protect the cardiovascular system against heart disease, and regulate cholesterol. This powerful antioxidant protects against cancer-causing free radicals.

How much do you need?
Recommended dosage is 500-1000 mg's per day. Many standard dosage amounts may be much lower so you can discuss this with your healthcare practitioner to see what's best for you. Getting too much is usually not a problem since any excess is eliminated via the urinary

tract. Because it's water soluble, Vitamin C does not get stored by the body. So getting C every day is crucial. It can be taken in large doses because what the body doesn't need can be easily eliminated because of the solubility.

How to get it:
While you can certainly supplement with a variety of C tablets, capsules, powders and chewables, I always try to get as much nutrition as possible from whole foods (in this case citrus makes the perfect choice). The reason for this is that I feel that vitamins in a whole food are much more beneficial than a pill, providing us with fiber and loads of other nutrients in a form our body easily and eagerly recognizes. (And when I say eagerly I mean it, I bet you right now if you think of an orange, or see one, you will start to salivate!)

You can still supplement to get that extra C, but by following the Vitamin C tips below, you can be sure to not only get your C but a host of other antioxidants, vitamins and minerals in a form far more delicious than any powder or tablet.

12 Ways to easily get 100mgs or more of Vitamin C

2 navel oranges (260mg)
½ large papaya (230mg)
1 large red pepper (209mg)

10 brussel sprouts (130mg)
2 little kiwis (128mg)
1 grapefruit (110mg)
2 large potatoes boiled and mashed (110mg)
3 cups steamed beet greens (107mg)
15 strawberries (105mg)
1 cup chopped broccoli (101mg)
½ cantaloupe (100mg)
4 tomatoes (i.e. raw, in a salsa or in a marinara) (100mg)

What are the signs of a Vitamin C deficiency?
Signs of Vitamin C deficiency include: dry or splitting hair, gum diseases, dry scaly skin, slow healing wounds, nosebleeds, and in severe cases, scurvy. It's easy to see what your daily intake is by using a food tracker like this one: www.cronometer.com, which is free and simple to use.

March - Food To Fuel Your Immune System

"Like any fighting force, the immune system army marches on its stomach."
- Harvard Health Publications

Scientists have long recognized that people who live in poverty and are malnourished are more vulnerable to infectious diseases. Whether the increased rate of disease is caused by the effects of malnutrition on the immune system, however, is not certain. There are still relatively few studies of the effects of nutrition on the immune system of humans, and even fewer studies that tie the effects of nutrition directly to the development (versus the treatment) of diseases.

When it comes to immunity, eating right is extremely important because the stomach is your immunity system's home base; its headquarters or 'Houston'. The entire digestive system, like all other bodily systems, is integral to optimal health. It is interconnected with your organs and the physiological needs of your entire body.

In short, what food goes in your stomach directly affects your immunity. The chemical processes that happen when you eat foods like deep-fried anything, fast food or chemical-laden processed foods, are *completely different* than when you eat a large salad and some vegetable curry.

What you decide to put in your body – the fuel that you choose - will directly affect your immunity. You have the power through food choices to improve your body's defense system. Most of us now have the knowledge, too, but the difficulty can be with implementing better eating habits. It's hard to change and reduce what we love to eat unless we can view these changes as opportunities to:

Try new dishes
A few days ago I saw a recipe online for a side dish with roasted vegetables, pecans and cranberries, and am excited to try it out. Only I'm going to make into a meal, not a side dish!

Get a chance to notice positive changes in our health
I challenge everyone here to add a big salad to your daily intake, every day for a week and see what changes are noticed. The natural minerals like calcium, manganese, iron and sodium, combined with the antioxidant Vitamins K and A, Vitamin C (and a bit of all the B's) and high fiber content are going to favorably affect your digestive system. Fried foods and boxed meals full of salt and artificial flavors are going to have negative effects. Maybe you'll notice an improvement in

regularity, or less stomach acid. These are things you can look forward to and directly control.

Reduce our food expenditures

Face it, while strolling through the grocery store you will spend a lot less money if you focus on purchases in the produce area. Going even further, you can grow a garden, or even forage for some foods. Eating better can mean spending less.

Experience a higher level of energy

The more you minimize or eliminate the unhealthy foods in your diet, and the more you include choices like greens, fruits and vegetables, the more energy will be freed up from digestive issues to address other bodily needs. Fruits and vegetables take anywhere from 30 minutes to 2 hours to digest, starches like potatoes, rice, pasta and bread take at least 3 hours to digest. Meat and dairy can take up to 24 hours to digest - think about the energy expenditure.

People who complain that they don't want to eat that many plant foods are missing out. The more of this stuff going in, the better you will feel.

So what is the best fuel for us? Our optimal fuel is based in high quality carbohydrates like fruit, vegetables and whole grains. To meet the smaller requirements of protein and fat (between 10-20% of total calories), including foods like nuts, seeds and avocados would be ideal.

Increase fresh foods and grains like brown rice or quinoa, and decrease the amounts of fatty and/or high protein foods (I say 'and/or' because many times high fat foods are also high in protein, like meat and dairy).

From reading my books you probably know I am a vegan. If you're not one, you may think I'm pushing the fruits and vegetables as part of my agenda to convert meat eaters. In actuality, I would be remiss in writing a book about the digestive system without mentioning these two basic nutritive goals:

Eat more fresh foods
Eat less flesh foods

Because I would be lying if I said this doesn't make a difference. I have experienced it myself. To me, it is undeniable:

The better the fuel the better you will feel.

And by viewing it this way, by focusing on the benefit of feeling better, you are doing something to improve yourself and it doesn't feel as hard to forgo that steak for a hearty soup.

Here's my diet plan:

I know how to eat well and I try to do this as much as possible.

Pretty general, right? I know what to do and I'm going to do more of it. It's that simple. That's all it has to be. You don't have to kill yourself giving up every food and trying new diets that promise quick results. I know personally that the more I focus on a plain old *eat good* policy, and the less I try to micromanage everything I eat, the easier it is to make better food choices.

So here's what I consider to be the top ten best foods for immunity and why they made my list:

Berries – Antioxidants; they have the ability to repair damage from oxidative stress and inflammation. Not to mention they taste great alone or in just about any recipe.

Greens – I don't have to explain why, do I? Minerals, fiber, B Vitamins - Greens makes you feel good! Eat them raw, put them in your smoothie, make a huge salad, steam them with lemon, put them in soup, etc. etc.

Bananas – Because they are the most accessible food in the U.S. You can get bananas EVERYWHERE. 100 calories a pop of pure yummy carbs plus Vitamins C, B2, B3 and B5, potassium, manganese and magnesium. The largest source of fuel in my diet today. I've eaten about 8-10 per day for over six years, usually in a big morning smoothie with berries.

Lentils – After fruit, this is my favorite fuel. Loaded with Folate and high in all the B Vitamins (except B12), lentils are also chock full of minerals including iron, zinc, copper, magnesium, manganese, phosphorus, potassium and selenium. Lentils can be simmered in curry spice (or a myriad of other ways) for a delicious hot meal alone or with rice.

Flaxseeds – We're seeing news about the many upsides to eating flaxseeds on tons of blogs nowadays and there are good reasons why: just a small amount of the oil or ground flaxseeds will give you 150% or more of your daily Omega 3 Essential Fatty Acids (EFA). The EFA's in flaxseed oil, also plentiful in eggs and fish oils, have been found in many studies to be superior to the animal versions because of mercury and processing concerns. Fresh fish oil will almost certainly have some mercury in it, and fish oil supplements are subjected to high heat, bleaching and other refining processes, leaving the supplement a far cry from its original source - not what I would coin, a 'superfood'.

Side note: Flaxseeds also make an effective egg replacer in baked recipes (grind 1T and soak in ¼ cup of water for a few minutes, then add to baked goods recipe).

Sweet Potatoes - Another one of those perfect foods, sweet potatoes are full of good carbs, with plenty of fiber, protein, vitamins (especially Vitamin A, C & B's) and minerals including manganese and copper). They make a sweet, warming meal even just on their own.

Pasta – Because it makes a meal that everybody likes and provides plenty of fuel for our bodies. You can also do most anything WITH pasta, slather it in marinara, make a cold salad in the summer or mix it with pesto. I love quinoa and rice pasta because they are gluten free and offer more protein than wheat.

Carrots – Perhaps the greatest snack ever; did you know that one carrot has over 400% of your daily Vitamin A? They are literally sold everywhere and are great to dip in hummus or just on their own.

Watermelon - I'll never forget the day my Mom, feeling flustered at trying to feed her vegan daughter during family get-togethers, sliced a watermelon in half, stuck a spoon in it and put it on my plate. It was perfect! in fact that type of 'meal' could just about satisfy most of your daily requirements including fiber, iron, calcium, protein, carbs, B Vitamins, antioxidant Vitamins C and A, and a slew of minerals. Maybe eating a half a watermelon sounds unusual or downright freakish to you, but let me tell you, after eating a water rich, not to mention fabulously delicious meal, you will feel an amazing sense of satisfaction to go along with your abundant energy.

I will end this section by mentioning a wondrous plant that can be considered a food, a spice and a medicinal herb: **Turmeric**. This amazing Ayurvedic herb is a digestive bitter, a carminative (facilitates elimination of gas), an anti-inflammatory, and a decongestant for not only the intestinal tract, but for the lungs and throat as well. If you can only do one thing in April to detoxify your immune system, take 1200 mgs per day of this powdered herb, if supplementing by capsule. You can also add a tablespoon to your favorite rice dish, add it to a pot of steamed greens, add into any soup recipe, or make a hearty tea with ginger (by simmering for 20 minutes, straining and drinking).

I am not at all saying that anyone should try to eat *only these foods*! And there are probably hundreds of foods that could grace this list. But it's a good start in formulating a base of nutritional powerhouses that contribute to digestive health and overall immunity. We can tack a list of these and other superfoods on the fridge to remind us to include more of them each day in our diet.

April - Effective Natural Cleansing

Traditionally, springtime has long been characterized as a time of cleansing - whether by implementing a deep inner cleanse or through the 'spring cleaning' of your home. This is the time of renewal, and with the warm months just around the bend, we are given a chance to focus on purification rituals.

Let's focus on inner cleansing, since we have just endured a long winter and our bodies are most likely in need of a total reset. The cold and flu season affects everybody - even if you did not get sick that much, your body was still exposed to many more threats and your immunity system has been working hard to defend against all the viruses and bacteria you were faced with during the dark months.

So what can do we detoxify our immune system naturally? Here are two ways:

1. By using alterative herbs to purify our blood. If an herb is an **alterative**, that means it cleanses the blood by enhancing the assimilation of nutrients, speeding up the elimination of metabolic waste, neutralizing excess acidity, and aiding in protein absorption. Alteratives have bitter principles

that activate and stimulate our liver delivering high nutritive content.

Incidentally, two of the most powerful alteratives are widely viewed as two of the most pesky weeds. People work hard to eliminate these tenacious herbs from their yards and gardens:

Dandelion and Burdock

If only they knew that the roots of these two humble plants could provide them each spring with everything their body wants!

Dandelion Root
While the dandelion flowers plague many a lawn connoisseur, the roots pack in numerous detoxifying talents. High in antioxidants, dandy root acts as a hepatoprotective - meaning it's able to prevent liver damage. It also contains one of the highest concentrations known of Kynurenic Acid, an amino acid that supports digestive function and bile flow, increasing the transport of toxins out of the body.

Traditionally Dandelion Root has long been used in liver and gallbladder disease and as a diuretic. It helps remove excess water and helps in the elimination of toxins through the urinary system. It also works as a blood sugar stabilizer, a mild laxative and blood pressure normalizer.

So how can you get the wonderful powers of this herb into your body this spring? Here are three ways:

1. Dig it up the roots, brush off the dirt, and steam or boil them as you would other root veggies like carrots, and eat. They'll taste a little more earthy and more bitter but your body will love it.
2. Dig up the roots, brush off the dirt, slice and dry in the oven at the lowest temp for several hours. Later, grind it up and make Dandy Root Coffee (just as you would make a pot of regular coffee, only substituting the ground, dried root)
3. Take the tincture. For a thorough cleanse and for those not able to harvest fresh dandelion root, take 10 to 15 drops of the tincture every day for the entire month of April. It costs only about $10.00 U.S. dollars to do your body a world of good.

Burdock Root

Do you remember the little prickles that insidiously attached themselves to your pant legs while playing outside as a child? Or, God forbid they got in your hair! Yes, these same little burrs, that were the inspiration for Velcro, are the signal that you have found one of the earth's strongest and most widely used medicinal herbs.

Burdock provides not one, but three ways to detoxify your body:

-As a diuretic, Burdock helps eliminate toxins and excess acids from your liver (via the kidneys).

-As a diaphoretic: this means it is sweat inducing, encouraging toxins to leave your body through your skin.

-As an antibacterial and antifungal. It accomplishes these tasks by providing inulin, a carbohydrate that does not get digested as other carbs, but rather it goes to your colon intact and provides food for all your good bacteria, causing them to function optimally.

Immunity is often said to begin and end in the gut. By supplementing with Burdock Root, you are providing food for your healthy bacteria, while enhancing your body's effectiveness in removing toxins.

Now you know what's coming! How does one take Burdock? Try one of these ways:

-In a stir fry. You will find burdock root a/k/a Gobo Root in most grocery stores. Soak it for several hours before cooking, then just add it to your stir fry as you would carrots or other root vegetables (usually cooking for 5-10 minutes).

-In a tea. Since you're dealing with a root, simply simmer your roots for 20 minutes and drink the tea, or the 'decoction' that you've made.

-Peel as you would a carrot (but all of it not just the outer part, so that you end up with thin slivers that dry quickly), dry in your oven at lowest temperature for 1-2 hours, then grind up to a fine powder in a coffee grinder. Add a tablespoon at will to your favorite soup or smoothie.

JUST REMEMBER - the very best times to harvest roots are in the spring and fall. During these periods the power of the plant is in the root system (in the summer the power is in the flower, or leaves).

So, what's the second way to detoxify our immune system naturally?

2. By taking herbs that cleanse the intestinal tract.

This method of cleansing your immune system encompasses herbs that specifically target intestinal health. Mucoid plaque, which tends to build up in our intestines, creates a slimy coating that prevents proper nutrient absorption, attracts parasites and slows digestion. Using herbs to target this plaque and get things moving again is the emphasis here.

There are two that I want to mention b
of their effectiveness in cleansing our in
tract and because they just taste good!

Slippery Elm

This herb can be found in powdered form (or capsules) in herb shops and natural food markets. In fact, Thayers makes a wonderful throat lozenge with Slippery Elm that soothes the throat while giving all the digestive benefits (great for kids' sore throats).

Slippery Elm is soothing to all mucous membranes and coats the intestines beneficially while working to relieve constipation and get toxins moving out. It does this by specifically acting on the nerve endings in the gastrointestinal tract and activating the removal of toxins. This herb also provides antioxidant and anti-inflammatory support.

You can add a tablespoon of Slippery Elm to a tea, a bowl of oatmeal, or your baked recipes.

Peppermint

Who would have thought that drinking a cup of peppermint tea every day could have such massive effects on our digestive system? Long known for easing post meal digestive complaints (see, "After Dinner Mint"), Peppermint calms the muscles lining the stomach relieving gas, and stimulating peristalsis, which helps cleanse the colon. This lowly mint also improves bile production encouraging more efficient digestion of foods and better elimination of toxins.

A cup of hot peppermint tea is a lovely way to start your day, and naturally cleanses your gastrointestinal tract, readying it for optimal digestion, nutrient dispersion and better immunity.

May - Enhancing Brain Function For Better Immunity

While reading blog posts and related studies online, I came to this realization: I don't need a medical study to prove to me that the brain is connected to the immunity system. But even though I come from a background of holistic health and have practiced natural health methods for over a decade, I still feel the need to provide proof in my books of certain information.

But the brain connecting to the immune system? How could it NOT? While there are some very interesting studies and there are actually arguments going on in the medical world about this concept, one really only needs to stop and ponder - how could the immunity system possibly function optimally without a healthy brain?

For my readers who are not as comfortable as I am with my sweeping health generalizations based on common sense and nothing more, I provide this quote from a study recently done at the University of Virginia: "In a stunning discovery that overturns decades of textbook teaching, researchers have determined that the brain is directly connected to the immune system by vessels previously thought not to exist. The discovery could have profound implications for diseases from autism to Alzheimer's to multiple sclerosis."

And for thousands of years, humans have been practicing techniques that target both the brain and the body. Healing therapies that involve mind/body exercises like meditation, yoga and tai chi have been shown to have a direct correlation to the level of inflammation in our body, thus having an impact on those with autoimmune diseases, where the body's natural line of defensive inflammation goes out of control. Not only can mind/body methods affect immunity this way, but they can do so in a relatively short period of time.

So, if we have an understanding that brain health affects our overall health, then what can we do maximize our brain function, and in turn, our immunity? Here are 2 Ways:

Brain Supporting Herbs, and Mind/Body Exercises

1-Brain Supporting Herbs

Rosemary: This is one of my all-time favorite herbs. Though I am a reputed killer of house-plants (even though I'm an avid gardener and wild crafter), I do bring my one potted rosemary plant in for the winter each year. Just touching the plant and smelling your hands is invigorating. Inhaling the essential oil of this herb has direct effects on your brain.

I could fill up ten chapters on the medicinal qualities of rosemary but will stick to the properties most linked to brain and immunity - antidepressant, analgesic (pain relieving), protective, stimulant, nervine and antispasmodic. Rosemary energizes and stimulates the central nervous system, clearing your head and improving your memory. It even acts in a similar way to that of dementia pharmaceuticals, only without side effects and adding in other positive attributes (like antifungal and aphrodisiac).

You can eat rosemary as a spice, make a cup of tea with it, or take a tincture daily. But your best bet with this herb is aromatherapy - using Rosemary Essential Oil. A 15-minute steam inhalation or just 10 drops in your bath is all it takes. Other medicines, both allopathic and herbal, must be digested before their medicinal qualities can affect you. But inhaling an essential oil goes quickly and directly to the brain.

Gingko Biloba
As one of the oldest known plant species, Gingko has long been respected for it's effects in memory improvement and blood disorders. Research today points to its ability to open up blood vessels and make blood less sticky, while also providing antioxidant support.

Frequently prescribed in Europe for dementia, Gingko increases oxygen to the brain, protects nerve cells and promotes nerve cell growth. 120 mg of Gingko Biloba taken twice per day is the standard dose.

CAUTION: Check with your health practitioner before taking Gingko, it can have negative and dangerous effects when combined with certain pharmaceuticals, especially NSAID's and blood thinners.

Gotu Kola
Used extensively as an Ayurvedic herb as well as in Chinese medicine, Gotu Kola quiets the nerves, tones brain tissue, and increases alertness. As stress can make us more sluggish, this is the perfect herb for relieving stress while energizing our brain.

Gota Kola, incidentally, works directly in supporting the immune system as well, as an anti-inflammatory, antifungal, anti-carcinogenic, vulnerary (wound healer) and antibacterial.

It also makes a good coffee substitute for those looking to ditch caffeine, but still in need of a morning wake-up drink. The powdered herb can be taken in a tea, encapsulized or in a tincture.

2-Mind/Body Techniques

Three Mind/Body Exercise for the Brain
(and the immune system)

#1 Take a Walk in the Woods (or at least among trees or nature). In this I have vast experience as I walk every day in the woods and every time it brings me peace and mental clarity. Reality tells me it's good for my body and my mind to do this every day. Science tells us this:

"University of Michigan researchers found that memory and attention improved 20% when people walked in a park versus an urban environment. Natural settings have a restful effect, allowing the brain to better process information, says study coauthor Marc Berman, a PhD candidate and psychology researcher. Busy surroundings—noisy traffic, colorful billboards, and throngs of people—clamor for attention and distract you. An iPod can do the same, so leave it at home to emerge calmer, more focused—and better able to tackle your to-do list."

#2 Combine Exercise with a Positive Affirmation
We all know that exercise increases brain health, and immunity for that matter, so I won't bore you by telling you to exercise (except the walk in the woods!), but what about enhancing our fitness routine by targeting our brains as we work out?

For me, a lot of times during exercise, I'm actually stressing or working logistics out in my mind. But when I plan a specific topic to think about while working out, it leaves me feeling even more energized than a regular old workout.

You can try one of these affirmations during your workout, either out loud if you're alone, or to yourself:

"I can achieve greatness."

"My body is healthy; my mind is brilliant; my soul is tranquil."

"I make smart, calculated plans for my future."

Or, make up your own affirmation, specifically designed for and relevant to you. Imagine the positive effects of combining these two powerful activities!

#3 Emotional Freedom Technique (EFT)
Termed as a 'psychological acupressure technique," EFT provides a quick and easy way to improve the energy flow in your head and chest. You simply tap specific meridians while using positive affirmations simultaneously. Here is a link to a short video exercise showing you exactly how to do it http://eft.mercola.com/. Every time I have engaged in this exercise I have felt

overwhelmingly energetic and clear minded directly afterwards.

June

Personal Empowerment & Its Effects On Immunity

When we talk about immunity, we often concentrate on our physical health but we all know that you can be physically fit and eat the cleanest diet possible and still have a compromised immunity system. If we are anxious or depressed, if we have too many negative thoughts or if we spend too much time worrying or feeling overwhelmed, it's certainly time to pay attention to our emotional health before it begins to seriously affect our body's defense mechanism.

One of the easiest ways to cultivate personal empowerment is by focusing on incorporating positive habits into your daily life. Most of these actions can become routine very quickly because once started, they immediately start causing positive benefits.

Which habits will help you the most? The answer is any action that you take regularly that helps your health. Here are four to start with along with their benefits to immunity and overall health:

Meditate:
If at all possible, first thing in the morning. When this was first recommended to me it was explained like this, "When you first wake up, your subconscious and your conscious are in communication; this is the only time of day when this happens." When you can be present during this time you are helping your subconscious do its job - working out the problems in your head.

If you are looking for evidence that meditation increases immunity, there are many studies to back this up. UCLA researchers discovered that HIV positive patients that meditated regularly showed a marked reduction in their CD-4 cell count. Other studies have confirmed that even weekly meditation caused an increase in antibodies.

In my own life what I've noticed when meditating daily is that I have better mental clarity and more feelings of joy. It feels like somehow this exercise opens me up to many more possibilities and makes staying optimistic easier.

Emphasize In-Person Connections:
In our world it is all too easy to depend on our virtual circles of friends. While the Internet has given us an amazing opportunity to know people all over the world, it's so vital to have those 'in-person' contacts. Friends we can see in 3-D, hug and talk to without that split second

skype delay - it's a whole other way of communicating and utilizes all our senses.

Nurturing your friendships off-line will enable you to have the best of both worlds - an online support system and those you look forward to interacting with in person. Two dimensional is not enough for all our human relationships. Sometimes it's easier and takes less energy or less planning to talk online than to meet someone in person, but we need to keep all our human ties open.

Give:
I'm not necessarily talking about giving money to a charity, though that would probably be money well spent. What I'm getting at here is to be giving in all your interactions. When we can be thinking of others and acting upon their needs, it comes back in spades. I know this personally - when I have given selflessly, I have reaped the most rewards. People smile at you more and are happy to have you around. The feeling that you've helped someone is one that builds you up, gives you higher self esteem and a better sense of well-being.

Goal Setting:
This may sound really simple, but I've found that the more time and energy I spend creating and working on realistic goals, and not on feeling overwhelmed or worried about trying to get so much done, the more productive I tend to be. Energy and time spent on worrying over

a challenge isn't going to help you actualize positive results. Time and brainpower used to think of and develop solutions gives you many more solid benefits.

When you make a goal for yourself and post it somewhere prominent so that you see it regularly, you will think about it more often and your mind will start conceiving ways to reach that goal, much more so than if you continue to concentrate on why that problem is causing you so much trouble.

I would like to close this chapter by giving you a title written by my friend, Sandra Leon. Sandra's book, "*Success and Happiness,*" can easily be on Amazon and is a comprehensive yet easy to read guide to forming positive habits. I used her book to create a morning ritual that includes meditation, goal setting, affirmations, etc. and have practiced it every day since reading her book. The outline she provides makes it easy to create something that works right for you.

Having a time set aside every day to practice things like gratitude and deep breathing have served me very well and I wake up every morning looking forward to getting out my journal and completing my morning ritual.

y - Deep Internal Healing With Calendula

In the prime of summer, our immunity system is usually at it's peak, especially in colder regions. We're getting all of our natural D, we're able to be outside more and get more exercise, and the availability of fresh organic food increases in many areas. So now that it is warm and sunny, it is the perfect time for some deep, internal, immunity cleansing.

You may be thinking green juices or water fasting. What comes to my mind first and foremost is the herb, Calendula. It's always a celebration when I see the first calendula blooms, usually here in July. This brightly colored herb is super easy to grow, self sows readily, and the list of its medicinal uses is far too large to be able to include everything here.

Calendula is already used extensively as a medicine internally and externally. We know that it was used as a plague deterrent in Medieval times and today it's anticancer properties are still being studied.

You may have heard about the powers of calendula in treating skin ailments as it's a major ingredient in commercial lotions and salves. I have a family member who, when enduring radiation therapy, told me that the only thing that made the burns feel better was a simple beeswax and calendula salve I had made for them.

This herb is very unassuming in appearance, even looking a bit weedy at times. But here's the short list of what it can do for your immunity system:

-High in flavonoids, Calendula acts as a powerful antioxidant.
-A leading antiseptic among herbs, it provides antimicrobial actions.
-It has lymphatic properties, meaning it encourages lymph drainage.
-As a vulnerary, it speeds up healing by increasing blood flow and oxygen in affected areas of the body.
-It's commonly used as an anti-inflammatory in digestive problems, ulcers and gastritis.
-Promotes purging of toxins by stimulating bile discharge.
-Seriously, this list goes on and on.

In a nutshell, Calendula, packs a punch with detoxifying, healing and toning powers for your organs and your immunity.

So how do you take Calendula? Here are three easy ways:

1-Make a tea with the loose, organic herb (or your own dried calendula flowers), a teaspoon or two per cup of boiling water. Cover and steep for 20 minutes. It has a lusciously fragrant scent that whether drunk in July or December, will remind you of summer.

2-Use the dried petals as a decorative on salads or cooked dishes (like you might use saffron). They add beauty to your dish and a digestive aid in the mix.

3-Take the tincture through July. 10-15 drops, 3 times per day. Tinctures are a great way to extract the most medicinal properties while preserving the herb for years.

August - Using Essential Oils For Optimal Immunity

I really looked forward to writing this chapter because I've been using essential oils for about fifteen years now and I have seen their powers. I have experienced lavender essential oil during a migraine and seen a reduction in nausea. I have smelled eucalyptus essential oil and instantly felt relief from a cold. I've been using essential oils in all of my cleaning products, bug sprays and herbal body care products and I know they work.

Essential oils are to me the concentrated power of the herb's essence and by smelling these aromas, the medicine in the plant reaches our brain far sooner than if it had been digested, drunk or taken under the tongue. Right to the brain.

The best part about essential oils is that most of them can be used for a multitude of reasons. Meaning you can use an immunity-supporting essential oil and also receive many other benefits, such as pain relieving, or toning of the nervous system, or insect deterrence. Having even just a few essential oils in your home gives you dozens of ways to improve your health.

Another reason I looked forward to this chapter is because essential oils are almost ALL antibacterial, antiseptic, antimicrobial, antifungal and astringent. They make it easy to take positive steps in increasing our immunity, and they make it so enjoyable - you can find the scents you like the most and stick with them - chances are they will be all you need for extra immunity help.

Here's my four favorite ways to use essential oils to boost immunity:

1-Lime Essential Oil In Your Bath
As a stimulant, a pain reliever and a respiratory tonic, Lime essential oil in your bath will create a rejuvenating treatment for your immune system. Add 10-20 drops while drawing the water and enjoy the multitude of medicinal actions, including analgesic, anti-depressive, antioxidant, antiseptic, insecticidal, sedative and tonic, to name just a few.

2-Massage Oil
What better to fight immunity than to have someone massage it into you?! Massage oils are not only therapeutic but easy to make - just use a small amount of almond, sunflower, grapeseed or coconut oil and add 15 drops of essential oil. Olive oil can work in a pinch but the others tend to have better absorption (less oily).

For an immunity massage blend, you could add five drops each of: <u>Mint, Lemon Verbena and Rose Essential Oils</u>, a mix that will help stimulate circulation, speed up healing and deter sickness.

3- Natural Antibacterial Spray

In most natural foods stores and online you can find little antibacterial spray bottles called "Thieves". It is named after a secret blend of essential oils that were used by thieves in medieval Europe so that they could freely pick-pocket the dead bodies of plague victims without contracting the horrible 'Black Death.' I say, if it worked for the plague, it ought to work for the viruses and bugs we have going around every winter.

The essential oils in the spray bottle are: **Cloves, Cinnamon, Lemon, Eucalyptus and Rosemary**. If you have a small glass spray bottle (you can also buy them pretty cheaply online), simply mix 1 part water, 1 part witch hazel (which can be found in any supermarket or pharmacy) and 5-10 drops each of the above essential oils. Now you have an all natural yet effective antibacterial spray for your home, your car, for work, or for the bathroom.

Added bonus: Because the witch hazel is an alcohol extraction, this spray will not freeze in your car, or anywhere outside.

Second added bonus: You could actually make this recipe using just one essential oil: Lavender - and be covered for air and hand sanitizing throughout the year.

4-Steam Inhalation With Eucalyptus and Peppermint

I'm not sure if there's anything more relaxing then a steam inhalation, and it's so easy to do right in your kitchen. All you need is a large glass bowl, boiling water, 5 drops of essential oil and a large towel. Pour the oils into the bowl first and then add the boiling water. Place the bowl at your table or desk, sit comfortably and lean your face over the bowl, covering your head and the bowl with the towel. The distance between your face and the bowl will depend on how hot the water is. Nothing should feel painful. Find the comfortable spot and then breathe slowly and deeply for about ten minutes. This is also a great time to meditate.

Why Eucalyptus and Peppermint? Well, firstly, Eucalyptus is a powerful antibiotic, respiratory tonic, decongestant, antiseptic and antiviral. Secondly, Peppermint is antimicrobial, antispasmodic, energy boosting and soothes the respiratory tract.

September

Fermented Foods For Gut Health & Immunity

In Chapter 3 we talked a little bit about the stomach being the headquarters for our immunity system. In fact it not only contains about 80% of our immune system cells, but it also houses our secondary nervous system and sports about as many neurotransmitters as the brain. In other words, the stomach is where it's at as far as getting healthier.

Luckily there are numerous food choices to directly and positively affect your own body's chances of avoiding sickness - and fermented foods are among the top picks.

When we have plenty of good bacteria in our gut, our digestion is improved and the fuel our bodies require gets to where it needs to go. The composition of our good bacteria, or our microflora, depends greatly on what food we give to it.

By eating fermented foods you are enhancing your digestion and exposing yourself to these many benefits:

1-An abundance of Vitamin K2 which helps decrease artery build up and heart disease
2-Stimulates the production of antibodies to pathogens
3-Acting as chelators, fermented foods draw out toxins and heavy metals
4-Offers an economical super food, you only need a little bit each day
5-By varying your fermented foods, you can vary the beneficial bacteria
6-You may even see an impact in your behavior, and experience a feeling of being more grounded

A few things are pretty clear. One is that when we take pharmaceutical antibiotics, which I would say are necessary in some extreme situations, they kill much of our intestinal flora, further weakening our system, when we are already sick. The second thing is that we can easily restore our system's microflora easily and deliciously. Here's 3 ways:

Kombucha - Have you tried any of this stuff? I am seriously addicted and it's a good thing. I've been studying how to make it and can't wait to finish my first batch. You may have heard of a kombucha mushroom. But there's no mushroom, only a mushroom-shaped, healthy bacteria-spewing 'scoby' that feeds off the sugar, tea and herbs you provide. In the resulting process you get improved, gut-healthy flora and loads of nutrients, all in the form of a delicious naturally carbonated drink.

Try some Gingerade Ginger Love Kombucha made by GTS - doesn't it sound like something you want to drink? You will be amazed at how good it tastes, it feels decadent and it's absolutely good for you. Or you can learn to make your own, there are several great YouTube videos breaking it down simply.

Keep in mind that while herbs and herbal teas can also be used in making kombucha, there needs to be some actual Tea in there, be it green or black, in order for the scoby to grow properly.

Kimchi - One thing that I love about Kimchi is that not only does the process of making it preserve the nutrients in the fresh vegetables, but it also produces probiotics to benefit your digestive and immune system. A second thing I like about it is that it's hot and spicy.

Kimchi may be added to any dish with rice, potatoes, tortillas or bread to make a flavorful meal that stimulates your digestion and pumps up your flora. You could also just have a little bit alone for a quick pick-me-up.

Traditionally, kimchi is made with a fish sauce, but for those vegetarians out there, water and flaked seaweed makes a perfect substitution. For a great kimchi recipe, check out this website:

http://www.maangchi.com/recipe/tongbaechu-kimchi

I would love to hear how yours came out. Also remember you can tweak the amounts of spices and red pepper to make it hotter or milder.

Raw Coconut Yogurt - Here it is, my latest not-guilty pleasure. As a vegan I'll admit there are many foods I miss; yogurt was one of them until recently. I stumbled upon raw coconut yogurt, sweetened with just a tad of vanilla, in the natural section of my grocery store; pure heaven. You can pick some up in a natural foods market or supermarket, or find plenty of web options for making your own.

One final note, probiotic foods are serious superfoods and a little can go a long way. You can have just a bit every day and your gut health will be better for it.

October - Winter Preparation Month #1

To me, October is a crucial time for thinking about winter health. For many of us, this is the time of year when it's getting colder, and much darker. The air inside our homes is drier, and we're probably spending less time outside. Just these few things can have a huge effect on our immunity. Luckily there are many ways we can support and prepare our bodies during this pre-winter time.

For October and November each I'm offering four natural ways to get ready for winter, a medicinal herb, a spice, a particular food and a mushroom. So let's start with October's:

October's Herb-Echinacea
Where I live, If you have a patch of Echinacea in a garden by a meadow, it's going to get eaten by deer. And do you know WHEN it's going to get eaten by deer? That's right, October. These gorgeous wild animals know exactly what to eat before winter and they set the example for their human counterparts. Thankfully, after grazing in the Echinacea patch, they will leave the roots, where the most concentrated medicinal properties lie. And during the fall months, the plant's powers are in

the root system and can be harvested and dried or tinctured for later use.

If you plan to harvest the flowers and leaves (all parts of this plant are medicinal), I would do that *before* October.

Personally I like to dry the herb and make tea with it combined with Peppermint and Mullein. Having a cup of Echinacea tea every day will give a huge boost to your immune system as you head into winter. How does it do this? By reducing inflammation and stimulating an increase in white blood cells.

By the time the 3rd week of October rolls around, and Daylight Saving happens in the U.S., our bodies, thrown off by an hour, (and being tempted by the candy extravaganza that greets us at every turn leading up to Halloween), have had just about enough. Inevitably this is when sickness hits our house. And if you have 3 weeks worth of Echinacea already in your system, I can tell you the symptoms will be reduced.

Since my Echinacea patch is small, and my harvest is usually gone quickly, I will often buy some bulk organic Echinacea for making teas throughout the fall and winter. I think the best way to take it is to drink the tea or take the tincture daily throughout October. And then supplementing when sick during the cold months.

So, do like the deer, and take your Echinacea in October.

October's Spice-Ginger
Of all the herbs I use, this may be the one I use the most. Yes, it's a spice to many. But its powers cannot be ignored. I love to make a fresh pot of ginger root tea as often as possible, especially in the fall. Here's why:

It keeps you warm -
It acts a natural analgesic
It's anti-inflammatory
It tastes delicious
It's antimicrobial and antioxidant
It inhibits the activity of cancerous cells
It contains natural antibiotics
It helps normalize blood sugar
It protects against respiratory viruses

So, whatever recipes you would normally use ginger in, just double or triple the amount of ginger. Or you can make a delicious, warming tea with a few tablespoons of chopped fresh ginger, boil for 15 minutes and drink.

October's Food - Pumpkin
Now I'm not just saying this because Halloween is this month and I'm jumping on the pumpkin spice bandwagon. Pumpkin is one of the healthiest foods sporting **14,100IU** of Vitamin A per cup of puree, a good amount of almost all the minerals (excluding selenium

and sodium) and at least 10% of your daily Vitamin B2, B5, C and E.

Vitamin A has been long associated with increased immunity and strengthened ability to ward off infection. Having a delicious food packed with Vitamin A plus all the other nutrients, fiber, iron and even a little protein as a staple during October is just plain smart.

And I haven't even mentioned the SEEDS yet! All the pumpkin information in this chapter has been based on the pureed or cooked squash. The seeds are basically a smorgasbord of nutrients. They have about the same amount of Vitamin A as the cooked squash, plus:

-Tryptophan isn't just in turkeys, folks. One ½ cup of pumpkin seeds provides 115% of your daily tryptophan.

-Over 100% of the following minerals: Copper, Magnesium, Manganese and Phosphorus, and 66% of your Zinc.

-Solid amount of every vitamin except B12 and D, being especially high in Vitamin C and Folate.

Pumpkin seeds (right from the pumpkin, or mechanically seeded) are great roasted lightly (300F for 15 minutes) with a bit of salt optional. They can be ground up and put into smoothies and baked offerings, or just eaten.

When we carve pumpkins in November, we always pick out the pie pumpkins (which sometimes come from our garden). Usually the large carving pumpkins are bred for size alone and the seeds (and puree for that matter) do not taste as good, and likely are not as nutrient packed as the pie pumpkins. But for fresh pumpkins, I like to roast the seeds whole, shell and all. They're delicious this way.

When you buy the seeds at the natural food market or online, usually they are just the hulled seeds, but these are still packed with nutrition and immunity boosting Vitamin A, etc.

October's Mushroom-Shiitake
While there are many exotic mushrooms that may have more immunity benefits than the shitake, I chose this one because of its commercial availability. Not everyone can identify a mushroom in the wild, and it's certainly not safe to do this without an expert showing you the ropes.

Luckily, Shiitakes can be purchased fresh in most western supermarkets or bought from natural food markets or online. Even if you can't get them fresh, they are readily available in bulk online and in stores in dried form.

Traditionally, this mushroom has been used for hundreds of years in Japan and China, usually steamed with vegetables, added into soups or just used as medicine. In modern times, studies have shown that Shitake mushrooms improve overall cell immunity.

Nutritionally, Shiitakes are rich in iron, B vitamins (especially B5), Copper and Selenium, and they also have a trace amount of Vitamin D.

Studies have concluded that these medicinal mushrooms help the immune system in two ways. They decrease the activity in an overactive immune system, such as in autoimmune diseases, and stimulates immune activity under certain circumstances. The polysaccharides in Shiitakes help to positively affect the immune system when it is threatened. In October, during the most difficult seasonal change, this is just what we need.

Saute shiitakes for 7-8 minutes to bring out their flavor and keep their nutrients intact. They are excellent in stir fries, omelets and I love adding a bunch to whatever soup I'm making or tossing a cup or two into a nice fresh marinara sauce.

November - Winter Preparation Month #2

November's Herb - Astragalus
Herbalists have long known the power of Astragalus in treating the immune system and tonifying the respiratory and digestive system. Astragalus circulates between the muscles and the inner skin enhancing the barrier against foreign invasion. In more recent times this herb has been shown to increase bone marrow's ability to make new blood, inhibit the spread of tumors and improve damaged lungs.

There's also been research that shows that taking Astragalus for the six weeks preceding flu season or allergy season has marked positive effects during this time. Supplementation can be done by taking capsules, tablets or a tincture. I like to buy the bulk root slivers and use in a tea when the months get cold.

November's Spice - Cinnamon
Most of us are familiar with sprinkling ground cinnamon in our baked goods recipes and delicious hot drinks. But as an essential oil, cinnamon gives you many ways of helping your immune system battle germs. By getting a small bottle of 100% pure Cinnamon Essential Oil (retails at about $6.00 U.S. dollars) in

November, you will have an early start in preparing for wintertime and the cold and flu season.

Used extensively in aromatherapy, cinnamon oil assists in the removal of toxins and blood impurities, improves circulation, reduces gas, stimulates appetite and lowers blood sugar. It also has anti-inflammatory, antibacterial, antifungal, antiviral, antioxidant and antiseptic actions. Internally and externally cinnamon oil helps your immune system protect against disease.

You can certainly buy an aromatherapy diffuser to spread the essential oil through the air but it is not necessary. Here are a few easy and practical ways to utilize the amazing powers of cinnamon oil during November, and straight through the winter:

1-Add 5 drops to your shampoo and/or conditioner. The steam of the hot water and the aroma will turn your shower or bath into a therapeutic treatment. By putting the drops into your bath, you are getting the external *and* internal benefits.

2-Make a simple air freshener by adding 30 drops of cinnamon essential oil and water in a spray bottle. Spray in your home, your bathroom, your car; anywhere you want. This can be repeated multiple times per day.

3-Put 3 or 4 drops on your scarf or in your hair and wear the essential oil all day.

November's Food - Blueberries
It's very easy for me to include blueberries in my winter readiness plan, because I live in the midst of enormous wild blueberry fields. I can get them fresh to freeze during the late summer and have a supply all year long. I can actually drive 20 minutes and buy 30 pounds of berries for about $60. any time of the year (just stop by Allen's Blueberry Freezer in Ellsworth, Maine). So, yeah, it's sure easy to include these in my daily diet and I have blueberries just about every day in my breakfast smoothie.

Many regions will also stock wild or cultivated frozen blueberries and it's great to have them on hand to provide your body with a megaload of nutrients. Their health benefits are mainly related to the antioxidant activity of the plant's Anthocyanins (the blue pigments) and there is some evidence that these pigments are a factor in fighting cancer and heart disease.

Nutritionally, they contain amounts of many vitamins including C, K, and B5, along with minerals potassium, manganese and copper. And face it, this food is delicious. Sprinkle some on your oatmeal, warm them up and just eat them (my kids love this), or feel free to add as many as you want to make your smoothie a delicious, nutritious, immune supporting meal - that's purple.

November's Mushroom - Chaga

I've had the pleasure in the past year to have a friend and neighbor introduce me to a new (to me) and utterly miraculous fungus: Chaga. My friend mentioned this to me last winter as she remarked that she hadn't gotten sick all winter, because she takes her Chaga every day. Since she mentioned that, I have talked with many others who have been harvesting it in my very town for generations. In fact, Chaga goes waaaay back. There's even a petrified mummy named "Otzi" that was discovered in the Alps in 1991 and believed to have lived around 3300 B.C. This mummy was discovered with a stash of what most researchers agree is the magical mushroom, Chaga.

Locally I see it on old birch trees near wet areas. It is said that the highest medicinal content of this mushroom is found on trees at least 25 years old. With Chaga, it's the older the better. Currently in Finland, the popularity of Chaga is immense, and its forests boast an estimated 4 million kilograms growing today.

So what is it about this mushroom that looks like a clump of blackened cottage cheese? This mushroom has not only been identified as the most nutritionally dense tree growth, but it also has been shown in studies over and again to stimulate the body's ability to heal itself.

Chaga contains betulin, which controls metabolic disorders, and betulinic acid which has been shown over and over again to be anti-tumor. Chaga directly aids the immune system by adding a multitude of antioxidants and acts as a potent anti-inflammatory. Inflammation is often the source of chronic disease so supplementing with Chaga during November helps to eliminate problems before the tough winter starts in earnest. Research done in 2007 concluded that Chaga has direct antioxidant effects in cases of HIV, IBS and Cancer.[9] There's even a story about a 12th century Russian tsar who purportedly healed his own cancer by taking Chaga.

If you're lucky enough to find Chaga in the wild, you can hack it off with a hatchet or chisel and hammer (it's as hard as the tree bark). Break it up into smaller pieces and dry it for a day in a gas oven with just the pilot light on (or in warm dry place for a week or so) until it is bone dry. Once dry, it can be grated and brewed just like coffee. Delicious! It does not taste like coffee, obviously, but it has it's own rich, earthy flavor and can be drunk daily during the month of November in preparation for a long winter.

December

6 Delicious Recipes For Immunity Boosting

Now we are in the hustle and bustle that is the Holidays. While we are preparing dishes to bring to parties and family gatherings, we can make a choice for immunity supporting foods and healthful beverages.

But we don't have to compromise taste when cooking with health and nutrition in mind. These six recipes are delicious to eat, wonderful to share, and will all boost the immunity system of those who partake. So we get to share some healthy and delicious food to counteract that peanut butter fudge and spiked eggnog!

Sweet Potato Casserole

Ingredients Sweet Potato Mixture:
5 large sweet potatoes peeled and chopped into chunks
3 T coconut oil
3 T maple syrup
1 t vanilla
¾ t cinnamon
⅛ t ginger

⅛ t nutmeg
salt to taste

Ingredients Crumble:
1 cup oats
1 ½ cup chopped pecans
⅓ cup ground almonds
1 T cinnamon
⅛ t salt
2 T coconut oil
2 T olive oil
¼ cup maple syrup

Directions:
Boil sweet potatoes for 15 minutes. Drain and mash with the rest of the sweet potato mixture ingredients. Spoon into a large casserole dish. Pulse oats a bit and mix with the rest of the crumble ingredients in a bowl with a fork. Sprinkle crumble onto casserole and bake at 375F for 20 minutes.

Creamy Mushroom Soup

With all the extra mushrooms you get a Vitamin D boost, and the other vegetables and herbs make this a tasty and warming crock pot entree.

Ingredients:
2 cups cauliflower florets
1 ⅔ cups unsweetened almond or rice milk
1 teaspoon onion powder
½ teaspoon black or cayenne pepper

2 cups diced shiitake, oyster or baby bella mushrooms
½ diced yellow onion

Directions: Simmer cauliflower in milk, onion powder, salt and pepper in a small saucepan for 10 minutes, until cauliflower is soft. Then puree this mixture and set aside. Sauteé mushrooms and onion in oil in medium saucepan until onions are translucent, about 10 minutes. Then add cauliflower mixture, bring to a boil and simmer for 10 more minutes. Ready to serve.

Basil & Garlic Pesto

At this point in the game, you probably already know that garlic has natural antibiotic properties, but you may have formerly considered basil only for its virtues as a spice. With it's high amount of Vitamin K, basil offers a potent immunity booster. This pesto is great with bread, pasta or for dipping veggies in.

Ingredients:
3 cups chopped basil
1 cup olive oil
½ cup pine nuts
¼ cup cashews
2 Tablespoons chopped fresh garlic
½ Tablespoon chile powder or cayenne

Directions:
Blend until smooth.

Vegan Pumpkin Pie With Coconut Crust

My favorite dessert, the toasted coconut crust makes me feel like a queen. But I didn't need a queen's kitchen maids to make it. Super easy and luscious, a dessert you can truly enjoy and never feel sorry for partaking.

Ingredients:

Crust:
1 ½ cup shredded coconut
3 T olive oil

Pie:
1 can pureed pumpkin (or about 10 oz of steamed fresh pumpkin drained a bit)
½ cup maple syrup
⅓ almond or rice milk
1 T olive oil
2 T arrowroot powder (or non-gmo cornstarch)
1 t ginger
2 t cinnamon
½ t allspice
couple dashes of nutmeg
salt to taste

Directions - Prepare pie crust:
Mix coconut with olive oil. Press mixture down and coat into a 8-9 inch pie plate and bake at 325F for 15 minutes, or until lightly golden.

Directions - Pie mix:
Blend all pie ingredients until smooth. Pour into baked coconut crust pie plate. Bake at 350F for

35 minutes. Should be firmish on top and may show a few cracks on the surface.

Feel free to top the pie with Coconut Bliss frozen dessert! YUM!!

Festive Salad
If you bring a beautiful salad with yummy ingredients, people will eat it, they will SCARF it, at least that's my experience. Feed the people with something good that looks amazing, it's a great way to go.

Ingredients:
1 10oz bag of mixed greens, or one head of romaine lettuce chopped
¼ cup diced red onion
1 cup chopped nuts (pecans and walnuts are especially good)
3 mandarin oranges/tangerines peeled and separated
1 pomegranate, seeded
2 Tablespoons balsamic vinaigrette

Directions:
Toss together the greens, onions, nuts and mandarins with the vinaigrette. Top with the pomegranate seeds.

Mulled Hot Cider
This recipes calls for lots of yummy spices that perform double-time as immunity boosters.

Ingredients:

6 cloves
2 cinnamon sticks
½ teaspoon allspice
pinch or two of nutmeg
⅛ teaspoon or less salt
¼ cup maple syrup
1 large orange, peel included, chopped
2 quarts of apple cider

Directions:
Put all ingredients (except the cider) into a cheesecloth ball, using ends of the cheese cloth to tie it up. Put the ball into a pot with the cider and heat but don't boil all ingredients for 20 minutes. Squeeze out the cheese ball and compost. Your cider is ready. Keep it in a crock pot to bring to a holiday event, and even garnish with some oranges slices and cinnamon sticks.

Bonus Recipe - One Last, Fantastic, Herbal Immunity Booster

Fire Cider!!
If you like doing shots, but maybe you don't appreciate the morning directly following shots, you could try a little fire cider. Tastes a lot like it sounds and will keep you warm on a winter day while helping your body fight disease at the same time. It feels like you're downing a shot of alcohol, but instead you get super medicinal herbs and foods to boost your immunity.

Ingredients:

1 chopped onion
¼ cup grated ginger
¼ cup grated horseradish
5 cloves garlic chopped
½ teaspoon cayenne
Apple Cider Vinegar

Directions:
Put first 5 ingredients in a large glass mason jar, or other glass container with a lid. Pour Apple Cider Vinegar over to fill. Let sit 4 weeks in a dark, cool place. Strain and add sweetener and extra cayenne to taste.

Conclusion

There are so many ways you can boost your immune system naturally. You certainly don't have to do all of them, in fact I'd be a little worried if you did. But having all these choices makes it easy to choose a few that work perfectly for you. I sincerely hope that you've drawn a few favorites from this book that will help strengthen your immune system for a lifetime.

Thank you for reading and being with me on my journey to better health.

More Books by Mary Thibodeau:

Ten Wild Herbs For Ten Modern Problems

Migraine: Natural Treatment and Prevention - The Holistic Guide To Natural Migraine Therapies

Immune System Boosters: How To Naturally Boost Your Immune System And Stay Healthy All Year Long

Cleanse: Holistic Strategies For Reducing Your Body's Chemical Load

Vegan: How To Be A Vegan In A Meat Eater's World – The Vegan's Guide To Thriving and Surviving

Healing Lyme Disease Naturally: The Handbook for Holistic Lyme Disease Treatment & Prevenion

References

http://www.huffingtonpost.com/2012/10/17/exercise-immune-system-t-cells_n_1971311.html

http://www.health.harvard.edu/staying-healthy/how-to-boost-your-immune-system

http://www.health.harvard.edu/staying-healthy/how-to-boost-your-immune-system

http://www.sciencedaily.com/releases/2015/06/150601122445.htm

http://ac.els-cdn.com/S0889159115001658/1-s2.0-S0889159115001658-main.pdf?_tid=a980e2b0-a8b7-11e5-abba-00000aacb361&acdnat=1450794428_5f1883bf80fe513a7550e284c57f679e

https://umm.edu/health/medical/altmed/herb/ginkgo-biloba

http://pss.sagepub.com/content/19/12/1207.abstract

http://www.chopra.com/ccl/how-meditation-helps-your-immune-system-do-its-job

http://www.faim.org/longevity/PPNF-Journal-Chaga.pdf

Made in the USA
Middletown, DE
21 June 2017